Ambulatory Surgery Center Regulation

The CMS Conditions for Coverage for Ambulatory Surgery Centers

2017 Edition

John J. Goehle, MBA, CASC, CPA
Chief Operating Officer
Ambulatory Healthcare Strategies, LLC

Published by:
Eden Group Development, Inc.
Spencerport, New York

Disclaimer:

V2017-090117

Other Books by John J. Goehle

Published by HC Pro

Financial Management Made Easy – Strategies for Ambulatory Surgery Centers

APCs for ASCs – Strategies for Success under the New Payment System

Published by Eden Group Development

The Survey Guide for ASCs - A Guide to the Conditions for Coverage & Interpretive
Guidelines for Ambulatory Surgery Centers

Ambulatory Surgery Center Governance - A Guide for Ambulatory Surgery Center Owners
& Governing Body Members

Medicare Regulations & Payment Policy for Ambulatory Surgery Centers

Selected Federal and State Rules, Regulations & Standards for ASCs

Table of Contents

Introduction

Medicare defines an Ambulatory Surgery Center as a "distinct entity that operates exclusively for the purpose of providing surgical services to patients not requiring hospitalization and in which the expected duration of services would not exceed 24 hours following an admission."

To become an ASC and bill the Medicare program and most other insurances, you must comply with the regulations established by CMS, as well as any state licensure requirements. In most states, you must be Medicare Certified to become licensed as an ASC within that state, even if you do not intend to take care of Medicare or Medicaid patients.

The Conditions for Coverage, issued by the Centers for Medicare and Medicaid Services (CMS) are the federal regulations that ASCs must meet to participate in the Medicare program and to obtain Medicare Certification.

These conditions (which include "standards" associated with each "condition") are updated periodically by CMS and those updates are published in the federal register. The conditions for coverage are broken into seven sections. This book contains an overview, a convenient index, and the complete text of the Conditions for Coverage.

Interpretive Guidelines for the Conditions for Coverage

The Centers for Medicare and Medicaid Services (CMS) provides guidance to State Surveyors regarding the interpretation of the Conditions for Coverage.

Revised guidance is posted periodically on the CMS website and the reader should check periodically for any updates. The web address for these updates is:

http://www.cms.gov/Medicare/Provider-Enrollment-and-Certification/SurveyCertificationGenInfo/Policy-and-Memos-to-States-and-Regions.html

When you load the site in your browser, you will want to search for "ASC" to bring up only Ambulatory Surgical Center Guidance.

It is highly recommended that ASCs review the guidelines and alerts as they provide an excellent summary of the rationale of the conditions and the accepted interpretation of their meaning. The clarifications are of particular importance given the focus survey teams tend to have on these issues.

The author publishes a companion to this book - The Survey Guide for ASCs - A Guide to the CMS Conditions for Coverage & Interpretive Guidelines for Ambulatory Surgery Centers which is available at Amazon or through the publisher's web site at www.reg-books.com.

Original Source Documentation

CMS maintains a web site that provides copies of the proposed and final rules as well as links to useful and updated information about the conditions:

http://www.cms.hhs.gov/CFCsAndCoPs/16_ASC.asp

The actual Conditions for Coverage are available through the Electronic Code of Federal Regulations Web Site (www.ecfr.gpoaccess.gov). The code is available through the following link and is reproduced in this book in its entirety.

http://www.ecfr.gov/cgi-bin/text-
idx?c=ecfr&rgn=div5&view=text&node=42:3.0.1.1.3&idno=42

Note that the Conditions for Coverage are not the only rules and regulations that an ASC must follow to maintain Medicare certification and State licensure. ASC administrators should consult their state laws for state-specific requirements. Also note that the Conditions for Coverage refer extensively to the Life Safety Code published by the National Fire Protection Association (NFPA). ASCs should have a copy of the applicable Life Safety Code for their facility – which is available from their web site at:

http://nfpa.org

Lastly, please remember to consult attorneys with a thorough understanding of the ASC industry prior to making important decisions regarding your ASC. No single online or written resource can provide you with the up to date regulatory guidance that you receive from a knowledgeable attorney.

Introduction

This section contains the complete conditions for coverage as contained in the Federal Register. See Part III for the interpretation of these conditions. Note that Part III is broken down by Subpart and Chapter just as the conditions for coverage contained herein.

The Medicare Conditions for Coverage for ASCs

Per the Federal Register as of June 22, 2017

Authority: Secs. 1102 and 1871 of the Social Security Act (42 U.S.C. 1302 and 1395hh).

Source: 47 FR 34094, Aug. 5, 1982, unless otherwise noted.

Subpart A—General Provisions and Definitions

§416.1 Basis and scope.

(a) Statutory basis. (1) Section 1832(a)(2)(F)(i) of the Act provides for Medicare Part B coverage of facility services furnished in connection with surgical procedures specified by the Secretary under section 1833(i)(1) of the Act.

(2) Section 1833(i)(1)(A) of the Act requires the Secretary to specify the surgical procedures that can be performed safely on an ambulatory basis in an ambulatory surgical center.

(3) Sections 1833(i)(2)(A) and (D) and 1833(a)(1)(G) of the Act specify the amounts to be paid for facility services furnished in

connection with the specified surgical procedures when they are performed in an ASC.

(4) Section 1833(i)(2)(C) of the Act provides that if the Secretary has not updated amounts for ASC facility services furnished during a fiscal year through 2005 or a calendar year beginning with 2006, the amounts shall be increased by the percentage increase in the Consumer Price Index for all urban consumers as estimated by the Secretary for the 12-month period ending with the midpoint of the year involved, except that, in fiscal year 2005, the last quarter of calendar year 2005, and each of the calendar years 2006 through 2009, the increase shall be zero percent.

(5) Section 1833(i)(2)(E) of the Act provides that, with respect to surgical procedures furnished on or after January 1, 2007, and before the effective date of the implementation of a revised payment system, the payment amount shall be the lesser of the ASC payment rate established under section 1833(i)(2)(A) of the Act or the prospective payment rate for hospital outpatient department services established under section 1833(t)(3)(D) of the Act. The lesser payment amount shall be determined prior to application of any geographic adjustment.

(b) Scope. This part sets forth—

(1) The conditions that an ASC must meet in order to participate in the Medicare program;

(2) The scope of covered services; and

(3) The conditions for Medicare payment for facility services.

[56 FR 8843, Mar. 1, 1991; 56 FR 23022, May 20, 1991, as amended at 71 FR 68226, Nov. 24, 2006]

§416.2 Definitions.

As used in this part:

Ambulatory surgical center or ASC means any distinct entity that operates exclusively for the purpose of providing surgical services to patients not requiring hospitalization and in which the expected duration of services would not exceed 24 hours following an admission. The entity must have an agreement with CMS to participate in Medicare as an ASC, and must meet the conditions set forth in subparts B and C of this part.

ASC services means, for the period before January 1, 2008, facility services that are furnished in an ASC, and beginning January 1, 2008, means the combined facility services and covered ancillary services that are furnished in an ASC in connection with covered surgical procedures.

Covered ancillary services means items and services that are integral to a covered surgical procedure performed in an ASC as provided in §416.164(b), for which payment may be made under §416.171 in addition to the payment for the facility services.

Covered surgical procedures means those surgical procedures furnished before January 1, 2008, that meet the criteria specified in §416.65 and those surgical procedures furnished on or after January 1, 2008, that meet the criteria specified in §416.166.

Facility services means for the period before January 1, 2008, services that are furnished in connection with covered surgical procedures performed in an ASC, and beginning January 1, 2008, means services that are furnished in connection with covered surgical procedures performed in an ASC as provided in §416.164(a) for which payment is included in the ASC payment established under §416.171 for the covered surgical procedure.

[56 FR 8843, Mar. 1, 1991; 56 FR 23022, May 20, 1991, as amended at 71 FR 68226, Nov. 24, 2006; 72 FR 42544, Aug. 2, 2007; 73 FR 68811, Nov. 18, 2008]

Subpart B—General Conditions and Requirements

§416.25 Basic requirements.

Participation as an ASC is limited to facilities that—

(a) Meet the definition in §416.2; and

(b) Have in effect an agreement obtained in accordance with this subpart.

[56 FR 8843, Mar. 1, 1991]

§416.26 Qualifying for an agreement.

(a) Deemed compliance. CMS may deem an ASC to be in compliance with any or all of the conditions set forth in subpart C of this part if—

(1) The ASC is accredited by a national accrediting body, or licensed by a State agency, that CMS determines provides reasonable assurance that the conditions are met;

(2) In the case of deemed status through accreditation by a national accrediting body, where State law requires licensure, the ASC complies with State licensure requirements; and

(3) The ASC authorizes the release to CMS, of the findings of the accreditation survey.

(b) Survey of ASCs. (1) Unless CMS deems the ASC to be in compliance with the conditions set forth in subpart C of this part, the State survey agency must survey the facility to ascertain compliance with those conditions, and report its findings to CMS.

(2) CMS surveys deemed ASCs on a sample basis as part of CMS's validation process.

(c) Acceptance of the ASC as qualified to furnish ambulatory surgical services. If CMS determines, after reviewing the survey agency recommendation and other evidence relating to the qualification of the ASC, that the facility meets the requirements of this part, it sends to the ASC—

(1) Written notice of the determination; and

(2) Two copies of the ASC agreement.

(d) Filing of agreement by the ASC. If the ASC wishes to participate in the program, it must—

(1) Have both copies of the ASC agreement signed by its authorized representative; and

(2) File them with CMS.

(e) Acceptance by CMS. If CMS accepts the agreement filed by the ASC, returns to the ASC one copy of the agreement, with a notice of acceptance specifying the effective date.

(f) Appeal rights. If CMS refuses to enter into an agreement or if CMS terminates an agreement, the ASC is entitled to a hearing in accordance with part 498 of this chapter.

[56 FR 8843, Mar. 1, 1991]

§416.30 Terms of agreement with CMS.

As part of the agreement under §416.26 the ASC must agree to the following:

(a) Compliance with coverage conditions. The ASC agrees to meet the conditions for coverage specified in subpart C of this part and to report promptly to CMS any failure to do so.

(b) Limitation on charges to beneficiaries. The ASC agrees to charge the beneficiary or any other person only the applicable deductible and coinsurance amounts for facility services for which the beneficiary—

For facility services furnished before July 1987, the ASC had to agree to make no charge to the beneficiary, since those services were not subject to the part B deductible and coinsurance provisions.

(1) Is entitled to have payment made on his or her behalf under this part; or

(2) Would have been so entitled if the ASC had filed a request for payment in accordance with §410.165 of this chapter.

(c) Refunds to beneficiaries. (1) The ASC agrees to refund as promptly as possible any money incorrectly collected from beneficiaries or from someone on their behalf.

(2) As used in this section, money incorrectly collected means sums collected in excess of those specified in paragraph (b) of this section. It includes amounts collected for a period of time when the beneficiary was believed not to be entitled to Medicare benefits if—

(i) The beneficiary is later determined to have been entitled to Medicare benefits; and

(ii) The beneficiary's entitlement period falls within the time the ASC's agreement with CMS is in effect.

(d) Furnishing information. The ASC agrees to furnish to CMS, if requested, information necessary to establish payment rates specified in §§416.120-416.130 in the form and manner that CMS requires.

(e) Acceptance of assignment. The ASC agrees to accept assignment for all facility services furnished in connection with covered surgical procedures. For purposes of this section, assignment means an assignment under §424.55 of this chapter of the right to receive payment under Medicare Part B and payment under §424.64 of this chapter (when an individual dies before assigning the claim).

(f) ASCs operated by a hospital. In an ASC operated by a hospital—

(1) The agreement is made effective on the first day of the next Medicare cost reporting period of the hospital that operates the ASC; and

(2) The ASC participates and is paid only as an ASC.

(3) Costs for the ASC are treated as a non-reimbursable cost center on the hopsital's cost report.

(g) Additional provisions. The agreement may contain any additional provisions that CMS finds necessary or desirable for the efficient and effective administration of the Medicare program.

[47 FR 34094, Aug. 5, 1982, as amended at 51 FR 41351, Nov. 14, 1986; 56 FR 8844, Mar. 1, 1991; 74 FR 60680, Nov. 20, 2009]

§416.35 Termination of agreement.

(a) Termination by the ASC—(1) Notice to CMS. An ASC that wishes to terminate its agreement must send CMS written notice of its intent.

(2) Date of termination. The notice may state the intended date of termination which must be the first day of a calendar month.

(i) If the notice does not specify a date, or the date is not acceptable to CMS, CMS may set a date that will not be more than 6 months from the date on the ASC's notice of intent.

(ii) CMS may accept a termination date that is less than 6 months after the date on the ASC's notice if it determines that to do so would not unduly disrupt services to the community or otherwise interfere with the effective and efficient administration of the Medicare program.

(3) Voluntary termination. If an ASC ceases to furnish services to the community, that shall be deemed to be a voluntary termination of the agreement by the ASC, effective on the last day of business with Medicare beneficiaries.

(b) Termination by CMS—(1) Cause for termination. CMS may terminate an agreement if it determines that the ASC—

(i) No longer meets the conditions for coverage as specified under §416.26; or

(ii) Is not in substantial compliance with the provisions of the agreement, the requirements of this subpart, and other applicable regulations of subchapter B of this chapter, or any applicable provisions of title XVIII of the Act.

(2) Notice of termination. CMS sends notice of termination to the ASC at least 15 days before the effective date stated in the notice.

(3) Appeal by the ASC. An ASC may appeal the termination of its agreement in accordance with the provisions set forth in part 498 of this chapter.

(c) Effect of termination. Payment is not available for ASC services furnished on or after the effective date of termination.

(d) Notice to the public. Prompt notice of the date and effect of termination is given to the public, through publication in local newspapers by—

(1) The ASC, after CMS has approved or set a termination date; or

(2) CMS, when it has terminated the agreement.

(e) Conditions for reinstatement after termination of agreement by CMS. When an agreement with an ASC is terminated by CMS, the ASC may not file another agreement to participate in the Medicare program unless CMS—

(1) Finds that the reason for the termination of the prior agreement has been removed; and

(2) Is assured that the reason for the termination will not recur.

[47 FR 34094, Aug. 5, 1982, as amended at 52 FR 22454, June 12, 1987; 56 FR 8844, Mar. 1, 1991; 61 FR 40347, Aug. 2, 1996]

Subpart C—Specific Conditions for Coverage

§416.40 Condition for coverage—Compliance with State licensure law.

The ASC must comply with State licensure requirements.

§416.41 Condition for coverage—Governing body and management.

The ASC must have a governing body that assumes full legal responsibility for determining, implementing, and monitoring policies governing the ASC's total operation. The governing body has oversight and accountability for the quality assessment and performance improvement program, ensures that facility policies and programs are administered so as to provide quality health care in a safe environment, and develops and maintains a disaster preparedness plan.

(a) Standard: Contract services. When services are provided through a contract with an outside resource, the ASC must assure that these services are provided in a safe and effective manner.

(b) Standard: Hospitalization. (1) The ASC must have an effective procedure for the immediate transfer, to a hospital, of patients requiring emergency medical care beyond the capabilities of the ASC.

(2) This hospital must be a local, Medicare-participating hospital or a local, nonparticipating hospital that meets the requirements for payment for emergency services under §482.2 of this chapter.

(3) The ASC must—

(i) Have a written transfer agreement with a hospital that meets the requirements of paragraph (b)(2) of this section; or

(ii) Ensure that all physicians performing surgery in the ASC have admitting privileges at a hospital that meets the requirements of paragraph (b)(2) of this section.

[73 FR 68811, Nov. 18, 2008, as amended at 81 FR 64022, Sept. 16, 2016]

§416.42   Condition for coverage—Surgical services.

Surgical procedures must be performed in a safe manner by qualified physicians who have been granted clinical privileges by the governing body of the ASC in accordance with approved policies and procedures of the ASC.

(a) Standard: Anesthetic risk and evaluation. (1) A physician must examine the patient immediately before surgery to evaluate the risk of anesthesia and of the procedure to be performed.

(2) Before discharge from the ASC, each patient must be evaluated by a physician or by an anesthetist as defined at §410.69(b) of this chapter, in accordance with applicable State health and safety laws, standards of practice, and ASC policy, for proper anesthesia recovery.

(b) Standard: Administration of anesthesia. Anesthetics must be administered by only—

(1) A qualified anesthesiologist; or

(2) A physician qualified to administer anesthesia, a certified registered nurse anesthetist (CRNA), or an anesthesiologist's assistant as defined in §410.69(b) of this chapter, or a supervised trainee in an approved educational program. In those cases in which a non-physician administers the anesthesia, unless exempted

in accordance with paragraph (c) of this section, the anesthetist must be under the supervision of the operating physician, and in the case of an anesthesiologist's assistant, under the supervision of an anesthesiologist.

(c) Standard: State exemption. (1) An ASC may be exempted from the requirement for physician supervision of CRNAs as described in paragraph (b)(2) of this section, if the State in which the ASC is located submits a letter to CMS signed by the Governor, following consultation with the State's Boards of Medicine and Nursing, requesting exemption from physician supervision of CRNAs. The letter from the Governor must attest that he or she has consulted with State Boards of Medicine and Nursing about issues related to access to and the quality of anesthesia services in the State and has concluded that it is in the best interests of the State's citizens to opt-out of the current physician supervision requirement, and that the opt-out is consistent with State law.

(2) The request for exemption and recognition of State laws, and the withdrawal of the request may be submitted at any time, and are effective upon submission.

[57 FR 33899, July 31, 1992, as amended at 66 FR 56768, Nov. 13, 2001; 73 FR 68812, Nov. 18, 2008; 79 FR 27153, May 12, 2014]

§416.43   Conditions for coverage—Quality assessment and performance improvement.

The ASC must develop, implement and maintain an ongoing, data-driven quality assessment and performance improvement (QAPI) program.

(a) Standard: Program scope. (1) The program must include, but not be limited to, an ongoing program that demonstrates measurable improvement in patient health outcomes, and improves patient safety by using quality indicators or performance measures associated with improved health outcomes and by the identification and reduction of medical errors.

(2) The ASC must measure, analyze, and track quality indicators, adverse patient events, infection control and other aspects of performance that includes care and services furnished in the ASC.

(b) Standard: Program data. (1) The program must incorporate quality indicator data, including patient care and other relevant data regarding services furnished in the ASC.

(2) The ASC must use the data collected to—

(i) Monitor the effectiveness and safety of its services, and quality of its care.

(ii) Identify opportunities that could lead to improvements and changes in its patient care.

(c) Standard: Program activities. (1) The ASC must set priorities for its performance improvement activities that—

(i) Focus on high risk, high volume, and problem-prone areas.

(ii) Consider incidence, prevalence, and severity of problems in those areas.

(iii) Affect health outcomes, patient safety, and quality of care.

(2) Performance improvement activities must track adverse patient events, examine their causes, implement improvements, and ensure that improvements are sustained over time.

(3) The ASC must implement preventive strategies throughout the facility targeting adverse patient events and ensure that all staff are familiar with these strategies.

(d) Standard: Performance improvement projects. (1) The number and scope of distinct improvement projects conducted annually must reflect the scope and complexity of the ASC's services and operations.

(2) The ASC must document the projects that are being conducted. The documentation, at a minimum, must include the reason(s) for implementing the project, and a description of the project's results.

(e) Standard: Governing body responsibilities. The governing body must ensure that the QAPI program —

(1) Is defined, implemented, and maintained by the ASC.

(2) Addresses the ASC's priorities and that all improvements are evaluated for effectiveness.

(3) Specifies data collection methods, frequency, and details.

(4) Clearly establishes its expectations for safety.

(5) Adequately allocates sufficient staff, time, information systems and training to implement the QAPI program.

[73 FR 68812, Nov. 18, 2008]

§416.44 Condition for coverage — Environment.

The ASC must have a safe and sanitary environment, properly constructed, equipped, and maintained to protect the health and safety of patients.

(a) Standard: Physical environment. The ASC must provide a functional and sanitary environment for the provision of surgical services.

(1) Each operating room must be designed and equipped so that the types of surgery conducted can be performed in a manner that protects the lives and assures the physical safety of all individuals in the area.

(2) The ASC must have a separate recovery room and waiting area.

(b) Standard: Safety from fire. (1) Except as otherwise provided in this section, the ASC must meet the provisions applicable to Ambulatory Health Care Occupancies, regardless of the number of patients served, and must proceed in accordance with the Life Safety Code (NFPA 101 and Tentative Interim Amendments TIA 12-1, TIA 12-2, TIA 12-3, and TIA 12-4).

(2) In consideration of a recommendation by the State survey agency or Accrediting Organization or at the discretion of the Secretary, may waive, for periods deemed appropriate, specific provisions of the Life Safety Code, which would result in unreasonable hardship upon an ASC, but only if the waiver will not adversely affect the health and safety of the patients.

(3) The provisions of the Life Safety Code do not apply in a State if CMS finds that a fire and safety code imposed by State law adequately protects patients in an ASC.

(4) An ASC may place alcohol-based hand rub dispensers in its facility if the dispensers are installed in a manner that adequately protects against inappropriate access.

(5) When a sprinkler system is shut down for more than 10 hours, the ASC must:

(i) Evacuate the building or portion of the building affected by the system outage until the system is back in service, or

(ii) Establish a fire watch until the system is back in service.

(6) Beginning July 5ʹ 2017, an ASC must be in compliance with Chapter 21.3.2.1, Doors to hazardous areas.

© Standard: Building Safety. Except as otherwise provided in this section, the ASC must meet the applicable provisions and must proceed in accordance with the 2012 edition of the Health Care Facilities Code (NFPA 99, and Tentative Interim Amendments TIA 12-2, TIA 12-3, TIA 12-4, TIA 12-5 and TIA 12-6).

(1) Chapters 7, 8, 12, and 13 of the adopted Health Care Facilities Code do not apply to an ASC.

(2) If application of the Health Care Facilities Code required under paragraph (c) of this section would result in unreasonable hardship for the ASC, CMS may waive specific provisions of the Health Care Facilities Code, but only if the waiver does not adversely affect the health and safety of patients.

(d) Standard: Emergency equipment. The ASC medical staff and governing body of the ASC coordinates, develops, and revises ASC policies and procedures to specify the types of emergency equipment required for use in the ASC's operating room. The equipment must meet the following requirements:

(1) Be immediately available for use during emergency situations.

(2) Be appropriate for the facility's patient population.

(3) Be maintained by appropriate personnel.

(e) Standard: Emergency personnel. Personnel trained in the use of emergency equipment and in cardiopulmonary resuscitation must be available whenever there is a patient in the ASC.

(f) The standards incorporated by reference in this section are approved for incorporation by reference by the Director of the Office of the Federal Register in accordance with 5 U.S.C. 552(a) and 1 CFR part 51. You may inspect a copy at the CMS Information Resource Center, 7500 Security Boulevard, Baltimore, MD or at the National Archives and Records Administration (NARA). For information on the availability of this material at NARA, call 202-741-6030, or go to:

http://www.archives.gov/federal_register/code_of_federal_regulati ons/ibr_locations.html. If any changes in this edition of the Code are incorporated by reference, CMS will publish a document in the FEDERAL REGISTER to announce the changes.

(1) National Fire Protection Association, 1 Batterymarch Park, Quincy, MA 02169, www.nfpa.org, 1.617.770.3000.

(i) NFPA 99, Standards for Health Care facilities Code of the National Fire Protection Association 99, 2012 edition, issued August 11, 2011.

(ii) TIA 12-2 to NFPA 99, issued August 11, 2011.

(iii) TIA 12-3 to NFPA 99, issued August 9, 2012.

(iv) TIA 12-4 to NFPA 99, issued March 7, 2013.

(v) TIA 12-5 to NFPA 99, issued August 1, 2013.

(vi) TIA 12-6 to NFPA 99, issued March 3, 2014.

(vii) NFPA 101, Life Safety Code, 2012 edition, issued August 11, 2011;

(viii) TIA 12-1 to NFPA 101, issued August 11, 2011.

(ix) TIA 12-2 to NFPA 101, issued October 30, 2012.

(x) TIA 12-3 to NFPA 101, issued October 22, 2013.

(xi) TIA 12-4 to NFPA 101, issued October 22, 2013.

(2) [Reserved]

[47 FR 34094, Aug. 5, 1982, amended at 53 FR 11508, Apr. 7, 1988; 54 FR 4026, Jan. 27, 1989; 68 FR 1385, Jan. 10, 2003; 69 FR 18803, Apr. 9, 2004; 70 FR 15237, Mar. 25, 2005; 71 FR 55339, Sept. 22, 2006; 77 FR 29030, May 16, 2012; 81 FR 26896, May 4, 2016; 81 FR 42548, June 30, 2016]

§416.45   Condition for coverage—Medical staff.

The medical staff of the ASC must be accountable to the governing body.

(a) Standard: Membership and clinical privileges. Members of the medical staff must be legally and professionally qualified for the positions to which they are appointed and for the performance of privileges granted. The ASC grants privileges in accordance with recommendations from qualified medical personnel.

(b) Standard: Reappraisals. Medical staff privileges must be periodically reappraised by the ASC. The scope of procedures performed in the ASC must be periodically reviewed and amended as appropriate.

(c) Standard: Other practitioners. If the ASC assigns patient care responsibilities to practitioners other than physicians, it must have established policies and procedures, approved by the governing body, for overseeing and evaluating their clinical activities.

§416.46   Condition for coverage—Nursing services.

The nursing services of the ASC must be directed and staffed to assure that the nursing needs of all patients are met.

(a) Standard: Organization and staffing. Patient care responsibilities must be delineated for all nursing service personnel. Nursing services must be provided in accordance with recognized standards of practice. There must be a registered nurse available for emergency treatment whenever there is a patient in the ASC.

(b) [Reserved]

§416.47   Condition for coverage—Medical records.

The ASC must maintain complete, comprehensive, and accurate medical records to ensure adequate patient care.

(a) Standard: Organization. The ASC must develop and maintain a system for the proper collection, storage, and use of patient records.

(b) Standard: Form and content of record. The ASC must maintain a medical record for each patient. Every record must be accurate, legible, and promptly completed. Medical records must include at least the following:

(1) Patient identification.

(2) Significant medical history and results of physical examination.

(3) Pre-operative diagnostic studies (entered before surgery), if performed.

(4) Findings and techniques of the operation, including a pathologist's report on all tissues removed during surgery, except those exempted by the governing body.

(5) Any allergies and abnormal drug reactions.

(6) Entries related to anesthesia administration.

(7) Documentation of properly executed informed patient consent.

(8) Discharge diagnosis.

§416.48 Condition for coverage—Pharmaceutical services.

The ASC must provide drugs and biologicals in a safe and effective manner, in accordance with accepted professional practice, and under the direction of an individual designated responsible for pharmaceutical services.

(a) Standard: Administration of drugs. Drugs must be prepared and administered according to established policies and acceptable standards of practice.

(1) Adverse reactions must be reported to the physician responsible for the patient and must be documented in the record.

(2) Blood and blood products must be administered by only physicians or registered nurses.

(3) Orders given orally for drugs and biologicals must be followed by a written order, signed by the prescribing physician.

(b) [Reserved]

§416.49   Condition for coverage—Laboratory and radiologic services.

(a) Standard: Laboratory services. If the ASC performs laboratory services, it must meet the requirements of part 493 of this chapter. If the ASC does not provide its own laboratory services, it must have procedures for obtaining routine and emergency laboratory services from a certified laboratory in accordance with part 493 of this chapter. The referral laboratory must be certified in the appropriate specialties and subspecialties of service to perform the referred tests in accordance with the requirements of Part 493 of this chapter.

(b) Standard: Radiologic services. (1) Radiologic services may only be provided when integral to procedures offered by the ASC and must meet the requirements specified in §482.26(b), (c)(2), and (d)(2) of this chapter.

(2) If radiologic services are utilized, the governing body must appoint an individual qualified in accordance with State law and ASC policies who is responsible for assuring all radiologic services are provided in accordance with the requirements of this section.

[73 FR 68812, Nov. 18, 2008, as amended at 79 FR 27153, May 12, 2014]

§416.50   Condition for coverage—Patient rights.

The ASC must inform the patient or the patient's representative or surrogate of the patient's rights and must protect and promote the exercise of these rights, as set forth in this section. The ASC must also post the written notice of patient rights in a place or places within the ASC likely to be noticed by patients waiting for treatment or by the patient's representative or surrogate, if applicable.

(a) Standard: Notice of Rights. An ASC must, prior to the start of the surgical procedure, provide the patient, the patient's representative, or the patient's surrogate with verbal and written notice of the patient's rights in a language and manner that ensures the patient, the representative, or the surrogate understand all of the patient's rights as set forth in this section. The ASC's notice of rights must include the address and telephone number of the State agency to which patients may report complaints, as well as the Web site for the Office of the Medicare Beneficiary Ombudsman.

(b) Standard: Disclosure of physician financial interest or ownership. The ASC must disclose, in accordance with Part 420 of this subchapter, and where applicable, provide a list of physicians who have financial interest or ownership in the ASC facility. Disclosure of information must be in writing.

(c) Standard: Advance directives. The ASC must comply with the following requirements:

(1) Provide the patient or, as appropriate, the patient's representative with written information concerning its policies on advance directives, including a description of applicable State health and safety laws and, if requested, official State advance directive forms.

(2) Inform the patient or, as appropriate, the patient's representative of the patient's right to make informed decisions regarding the patient's care.

(3) Document in a prominent part of the patient's current medical record, whether or not the individual has executed an advance directive.

(d) Standard: Submission and investigation of grievances. The ASC must establish a grievance procedure for documenting the existence, submission, investigation, and disposition of a patient's written or verbal grievance to the ASC. The following criteria must be met:

(1) All alleged violations/grievances relating, but not limited to, mistreatment, neglect, verbal, mental, sexual, or physical abuse, must be fully documented.

(2) All allegations must be immediately reported to a person in authority in the ASC.

(3) Only substantiated allegations must be reported to the State authority or the local authority, or both.

(4) The grievance process must specify timeframes for review of the grievance and the provisions of a response.

(5) The ASC, in responding to the grievance, must investigate all grievances made by a patient, the patient's representative, or the patient's surrogate regarding treatment or care that is (or fails to be) furnished.

(6) The ASC must document how the grievance was addressed, as well as provide the patient, the patient's representative, or the patient's surrogate with written notice of its decision. The decision must contain the name of an ASC contact person, the steps taken to investigate the grievance, the result of the grievance process and the date the grievance process was completed.

(e) Standard: Exercise of rights and respect for property and person. (1) The patient has the right to the following:

(i) Be free from any act of discrimination or reprisal.

(ii) Voice grievances regarding treatment or care that is (or fails to be) provided.

(iii) Be fully informed about a treatment or procedure and the expected outcome before it is performed.

(2) If a patient is adjudged incompetent under applicable State laws by a court of proper jurisdiction, the rights of the patient are exercised by the person appointed under State law to act on the patient's behalf.

(3) If a State court has not adjudged a patient incompetent, any legal representative or surrogate designated by the patient in accordance with State law may exercise the patient's rights to the extent allowed by State law.

(f) Standard: Privacy and safety. The patient has the right to—

(1) Personal privacy.

(2) Receive care in a safe setting.

(3) Be free from all forms of abuse or harassment.

(g) Standard: Confidentiality of clinical records. The ASC must comply with the Department's rules for the privacy and security of individually identifiable health information, as specified at 45 CFR parts 160 and 164.

[73 FR 68812, Nov. 18, 2008, as amended at 76 FR 65889, Oct. 24, 2011]

§416.51 Conditions for coverage—Infection control.

The ASC must maintain an infection control program that seeks to minimize infections and communicable diseases.

(a) Standard: Sanitary environment. The ASC must provide a functional and sanitary environment for the provision of surgical services by adhering to professionally acceptable standards of practice.

(b) Standard: Infection control program. The ASC must maintain an ongoing program designed to prevent, control, and investigate infections and communicable diseases. In addition, the infection control and prevention program must include documentation that the ASC has considered, selected, and implemented nationally recognized infection control guidelines. The program is—

(1) Under the direction of a designated and qualified professional who has training in infection control;

(2) An integral part of the ASC's quality assessment and performance improvement program; and

(3) Responsible for providing a plan of action for preventing, identifying, and managing infections and communicable diseases and for immediately implementing corrective and preventive measures that result in improvement.

[73 FR 68813, Nov. 18, 2008]

§416.52 Conditions for coverage—Patient admission, assessment and discharge.

The ASC must ensure each patient has the appropriate pre-surgical and post-surgical assessments completed and that all elements of the discharge requirements are completed.

(a) Standard: Admission and pre-surgical assessment. (1) Not more than 30 days before the date of the scheduled surgery, each patient must have a comprehensive medical history and physical assessment completed by a physician (as defined in section 1861(r) of the Act) or other qualified practitioner in accordance with applicable State health and safety laws, standards of practice, and ASC policy.

(2) Upon admission, each patient must have a pre-surgical assessment completed by a physician or other qualified practitioner in accordance with applicable State health and safety laws, standards of practice, and ASC policy that includes, at a minimum, an updated medical record entry documenting an examination for any changes in the patient's condition since completion of the most recently documented medical history and physical assessment, including documentation of any allergies to drugs and biologicals.

(3) The patient's medical history and physical assessment must be placed in the patient's medical record prior to the surgical procedure.

(b) Standard: Post-surgical assessment. (1) The patient's post-surgical condition must be assessed and documented in the medical record by a physician, other qualified practitioner, or a registered nurse with, at a minimum, post-operative care experience in accordance with applicable State health and safety laws, standards of practice, and ASC policy.

(2) Post-surgical needs must be addressed and included in the discharge notes.

(c) Standard: Discharge. The ASC must—

(1) Provide each patient with written discharge instructions and overnight supplies. When appropriate, make a followup appointment with the physician, and ensure that all patients are informed, either in advance of their surgical procedure or prior to leaving the ASC, of their prescriptions, post-operative instructions and physician contact information for follow-up care.

(2) Ensure each patient has a discharge order, signed by the physician who performed the surgery or procedure in accordance with applicable State health and safety laws, standards of practice, and ASC policy.

(3) Ensure all patients are discharged in the company of a responsible adult, except those patients exempted by the attending physician.

[73 FR 68813, Nov. 18, 2008]

§416.54 Conditions for coverage—Emergency preparedness.

The Ambulatory Surgical Center (ASC) must comply with all applicable Federal, State, and local emergency preparedness requirements. The ASC must establish and maintain an emergency preparedness program that meets the requirements of this section. The emergency preparedness program must include, but not be limited to, the following elements:

(a) Emergency plan. The ASC must develop and maintain an emergency preparedness plan that must be reviewed, and updated at least annually. The plan must do the following:

(1) Be based on and include a documented, facility-based and community-based risk assessment, utilizing an all-hazards approach.

(2) Include strategies for addressing emergency events identified by the risk assessment.

(3) Address patient population, including, but not limited to, the type of services the ASC has the ability to provide in an emergency; and continuity of operations, including delegations of authority and succession plans.

(4) Include a process for cooperation and collaboration with local, tribal, regional, State, and Federal emergency preparedness officials' efforts to maintain an integrated response during a disaster or emergency situation, including documentation of the ASC's efforts to contact such officials and, when applicable, of its participation in collaborative and cooperative planning efforts.

(b) Policies and procedures. The ASC must develop and implement emergency preparedness policies and procedures, based on the emergency plan set forth in paragraph (a) of this section, risk assessment at paragraph (a)(1) of this section, and the communication plan at paragraph (c) of this section. The policies and procedures must be reviewed and updated at least annually. At a minimum, the policies and procedures must address the following:

(1) A system to track the location of on-duty staff and sheltered patients in the ASC's care during an emergency. If on-duty staff or sheltered patients are relocated during the emergency, the ASC must document the specific name and location of the receiving facility or other location.

(2) Safe evacuation from the ASC, which includes the following:

(i) Consideration of care and treatment needs of evacuees.

(ii) Staff responsibilities.

(iii) Transportation.

(iv) Identification of evacuation location(s).

(v) Primary and alternate means of communication with external sources of assistance.

(3) A means to shelter in place for patients, staff, and volunteers who remain in the ASC.

(4) A system of medical documentation that does the following:

(i) Preserves patient information.

(ii) Protects confidentiality of patient information.

(iii) Secures and maintains the availability of records.

(5) The use of volunteers in an emergency and other staffing strategies, including the process and role for integration of State and Federally designated health care professionals to address surge needs during an emergency.

(6) The role of the ASC under a waiver declared by the Secretary, in accordance with section 1135 of the Act, in the provision of care and treatment at an alternate care site identified by emergency management officials.

(c) Communication plan. The ASC must develop and maintain an emergency preparedness communication plan that complies with Federal, State, and local laws and must be reviewed and updated at least annually. The communication plan must include all of the following:

(1) Names and contact information for the following:

(i) Staff.

(ii) Entities providing services under arrangement.

(iii) Patients' physicians.

(iv) Volunteers.

(2) Contact information for the following:

(i) Federal, State, tribal, regional, and local emergency preparedness staff.

(ii) Other sources of assistance.

(3) Primary and alternate means for communicating with the following:

(i) ASC's staff.

(ii) Federal, State, tribal, regional, and local emergency management agencies.

(4) A method for sharing information and medical documentation for patients under the ASC's care, as necessary, with other health care providers to maintain continuity of care.

(5) A means, in the event of an evacuation, to release patient information as permitted under 45 CFR 164.510(b)(1)(ii).

(6) A means of providing information about the general condition and location of patients under the facility's care as permitted under 45 CFR 164.510(b)(4).

(7) A means of providing information about the ASC's needs, and its ability to provide assistance, to the authority having jurisdiction, the Incident Command Center, or designee.

(d) Training and testing. The ASC must develop and maintain an emergency preparedness training and testing program that is based on the emergency plan set forth in paragraph (a) of this section, risk assessment at paragraph (a)(1) of this section, policies and procedures at paragraph (b) of this section, and the communication plan at paragraph (c) of this section. The training and testing program must be reviewed and updated at least annually.

(1) Training program. The ASC must do all of the following:

(i) Initial training in emergency preparedness policies and procedures to all new and existing staff, individuals providing on-site services under arrangement, and volunteers, consistent with their expected roles.

(ii) Provide emergency preparedness training at least annually.

(iii) Maintain documentation of all emergency preparedness training.

(iv) Demonstrate staff knowledge of emergency procedures.

(2) Testing. The ASC must conduct exercises to test the emergency plan at least annually. The ASC must do the following:

(i) Participate in a full-scale exercise that is community-based or when a community-based exercise is not accessible, individual, facility-based. If the ASC experiences an actual natural or man-made emergency that requires activation of the emergency plan, the ASC is exempt -from engaging in a community-based or individual, facility-based full-scale exercise for 1 year following the onset of the actual event.

(ii) Conduct an additional exercise that may include, but is not limited to the following:

(A) A second full-scale exercise that is individual, facility-based.

(B) A tabletop exercise that includes a group discussion led by a facilitator, using narrated, clinically relevant emergency scenario, and a set of problem statements, directed messages, or prepared questions designed to challenge an emergency plan.

(iii) Analyze the ASC's response to and maintain documentation of all drills, tabletop exercises, and emergency events and revise the ASC's emergency plan, as needed.

(e) Integrated healthcare systems. If an ASC is part of a healthcare system consisting of multiple separately certified healthcare facilities that elects to have a unified and integrated emergency preparedness program, the ASC may choose to participate in the healthcare system's coordinated emergency preparedness program. If elected, the unified and integrated emergency preparedness program must—

(1) Demonstrate that each separately certified facility within the system actively participated in the development of the unified and integrated emergency preparedness program.

(2) Be developed and maintained in a manner that takes into account each separately certified facility's unique circumstances, patient populations, and services offered.

(3) Demonstrate that each separately certified facility is capable of actively using the unified and integrated emergency preparedness program and is in compliance.

(4) Include a unified and integrated emergency plan that meets the requirements of paragraphs (a)(2), (3), and (4) of this section. The unified and integrated emergency plan must also be based on and include the following:

(i) A documented community-based risk assessment, utilizing an all-hazards approach.

(ii) A documented individual facility-based risk assessment for each separately certified facility within the health system, utilizing an all-hazards approach.

(5) Include integrated policies and procedures that meet the requirements set forth in paragraph (b) of this section, a coordinated communication plan and training and testing programs that meet the requirements of paragraphs (c) and (d) of this section, respectively.

[81 FR 64022, Sept. 16, 2016]

Subpart D—Scope of Benefits for Services Furnished Before January 1, 2008

§416.60 General rules.

(a) The services payable under this part are facility services furnished to Medicare beneficiaries, by a participating facility, in connection with covered surgical procedures specified in §416.65.

(b) The surgical procedures, including all preoperative and post-operative services that are performed by a physician, are covered as physician services under part 410 of this chapter.

[56 FR 8844, Mar. 1, 1991]

§416.61 Scope of facility services.

(a) Included services. Facility services include, but are not limited to—

(1) Nursing, technician, and related services;

(2) Use of the facilities where the surgical procedures are performed;

(3) Drugs, biologicals, surgical dressings, supplies, splints, casts, and appliances and equipment directly related to the provision of surgical procedures;

(4) Diagnostic or therapeutic services or items directly related to the provision of a surgical procedure;

(5) Administrative, recordkeeping and housekeeping items and services; and

(6) Materials for anesthesia.

(7) Intra-ocular lenses (IOLs).

(8) Supervision of the services of an anesthetist by the operating surgeon.

(b) Excluded services. Facility services do not include items and services for which payment may be made under other provisions of part 405 of this chapter, such as physicians' services, laboratory, X-ray or diagnostic procedures (other than those directly related to performance of the surgical procedure), prosthetic devices (except IOLs), ambulance services, leg, arm, back and neck braces, artificial limbs, and durable medical equipment for use in the patient's home. In addition, they do not include anesthetist services furnished on or after January 1, 1989.

[56 FR 8844, Mar. 1, 1991, as amended at 57 FR 33899, July 31, 1992]

§416.65   Covered surgical procedures.

Effective for services furnished before January 1, 2008, covered surgical procedures are those procedures that meet the standards described in paragraphs (a) and (b) of this section and are included in the list published in accordance with paragraph (c) of this section.

(a) General standards. Covered surgical procedures are those surgical and other medical procedures that—

(1) Are commonly performed on an inpatient basis in hospitals, but may be safely performed in an ASC;

(2) Are not of a type that are commonly performed, or that may be safely performed, in physicians' offices;

(3) Are limited to those requiring a dedicated operating room (or suite), and generally requiring a post-operative recovery room or short-term (not overnight) convalescent room; and

(4) Are not otherwise excluded under §411.15 of this chapter.

(b) Specific standards. (1) Covered surgical procedures are limited to those that do not generally exceed—

(i) A total of 90 minutes operating time; and

(ii) A total of 4 hours recovery or convalescent time.

(2) If the covered surgical procedures require anesthesia, the anesthesia must be—

(i) Local or regional anesthesia; or

(ii) General anesthesia of 90 minutes or less duration.

(3) Covered surgical procedures may not be of a type that—

(i) Generally result in extensive blood loss;

(ii) Require major or prolonged invasion of body cavities;

(iii) Directly involve major blood vessels; or

(iv) Are generally emergency or life-threatening in nature.

(c) Publication of covered procedures. CMS will publish in the Federal Register a list of covered surgical procedures and revisions as appropriate.

[47 FR 34094, Aug. 5, 1982, as amended at 71 FR 68226, Nov. 24, 2006]

§416.75 Performance of listed surgical procedures on an inpatient hospital basis.

The inclusion of any procedure as a covered surgical procedure under §416.65 does not preclude its coverage in an inpatient hospital setting under Medicare.

§416.76 Applicability.

The provisions of this subpart apply to facility services furnished before January 1, 2008.

[71 FR 68226, Nov. 24, 2006]

Subpart E—Prospective Payment System for Facility Services Furnished Before January 1, 2008

§416.120 Basis for payment.

The basis for payment depends on where the services are furnished.

(a) Hospital outpatient department. Payment is in accordance with part 419 of this chapter.

(b) [Reserved]

(c) ASC—(1) General rule. Payment is based on a prospectively determined rate. This rate covers the cost of services such as supplies, nursing services, equipment, etc., as specified in §416.61. The rate does not cover physician services or other medical services covered under part 410 of this chapter (for example, X-ray services or laboratory services) which are not directly related to the performance of the surgical procedures. Those services may be billed separately and paid on a reasonable charge basis.

(2) Single and multiple surgical procedures. (i) If one covered surgical procedure is furnished to a beneficiary in an operative session, payment is based on the prospectively determined rate for that procedure.

(ii) If more than one surgical procedure is furnished in a single operative session, payment is based on—

(A) The full rate for the procedure with the highest prospectively determined rate; and

(B) One half of the prospectively determined rate for each of the other procedures.

(3) Deductibles and coinsurance. Part B deductible and coinsurance amounts apply as specified in §410.152 (a) and (i) of this chapter.

[56 FR 8844, Mar. 1, 1991; 56 FR 23022, May 20, 1991, as amended at 71 FR 68226, Nov. 24, 2006]

§416.121 Applicability.

The provisions of this subpart apply to facility services furnished before January 1, 2008.

[71 FR 68226, Nov. 24, 2006]

§416.125 ASC facility services payment rate.

(a) The payment rate is based on a prospectively determined standard overhead amount per procedure derived from an estimate of the costs incurred by ambulatory surgical centers generally in providing services furnished in connection with the performance of that procedure.

(b) The payment must be substantially less than would have been paid under the program if the procedure had been performed on an inpatient basis in a hospital.

(c) For services furnished on or after January 1, 2007, and before the effective date of implementation of a revised payment system, the ASC payment rate for a surgical procedure is the lesser of the ASC payment rate established under paragraph (a) of this section or the prospective payment rate for the procedure established under §419.32 of this chapter. The lesser payment amount is determined prior to application of any geographic adjustment.

[56 FR 8844, Mar. 1, 1991, as amended at 71 FR 68226, Nov. 24, 2006]

§416.130 Publication of revised payment methodologies.

Whenever CMS proposes to revise the payment rate for ASCs, CMS publishes a notice in the Federal Register describing the revision. The notice also explains the basis on which the rates were established. After reviewing public comments, CMS publishes a notice establishing the rates authorized by this section. In setting these rates, CMS may adopt reasonable classifications of facilities and may establish different rates for different types of surgical procedures.

[47 FR 34094, Aug. 5, 1982, as amended at 56 FR 8844, Mar. 1, 1991]

§416.140 Surveys.

(a) Timing, purpose, and procedures. (1) No more often than once a year, CMS conducts a survey of a randomly selected sample of participating ASCs to collect data for analysis or reevaluation of payment rates.

(2) CMS notifies the selected ASCs by mail of their selection and of the form and content of the report the ASCs are required to submit within 60 days of the notice.

(3) If the facility does not submit an adequate report in response to CMS's survey request, CMS may terminate the agreement to participate in the Medicare program as an ASC.

(4) CMS may grant a 30-day postponement of the due date for the survey report if it determines that the facility has demonstrated good cause for the delay.

(b) Requirements for ASCs. ASCs must—

(1) Maintain adequate financial records, in the form and containing the data required by CMS, to allow determination of the payment rates for covered surgical procedures furnished to Medicare beneficiaries under this subpart.

(2) Within 60 days of a request from CMS submit, in the form and detail as may be required by CMS, a report of—

(i) Their operations, including the allowable costs actually incurred for the period and the actual number and kinds of surgical procedures furnished during the period; and

(ii) Their customary charges for each surgical procedure furnished for the period.

[47 FR 34094, Aug. 5, 1982, as amended at 56 FR 8845, Mar. 1, 1991]

Subpart F—Coverage, Scope of ASC Services, and Prospective Payment System for ASC Services Furnished on or After January 1, 2008

Source: 72 FR 42545, Aug. 2, 2007, unless otherwise noted.

§416.160 Basis and scope.

(a) Statutory basis. (1) Section 1833(i)(2)(D) of the Act requires the Secretary to implement a revised payment system for payment of surgical services furnished in ASCs. The statute requires that, in the year such system is implemented, the system shall be designed to result in the same amount of aggregate expenditures for such services as would be made if there was no requirement for a revised payment system. The revised payment system shall be implemented no earlier than January 1, 2006, and no later than January 1, 2008. The statute provides that the Secretary may implement a reduction in any annual update for failure to report on quality measures as specified by the Secretary. The statute also requires that, for CY 2011 and each subsequent year, any annual update to the ASC payment system, after application of any reduction in the annual update for failure to report on quality measures as specified by the Secretary, be reduced by a productivity adjustment. There shall be no administrative or judicial review under section 1869 of the Act, section 1878 of the Act, or otherwise of the classification system, the relative weights, payment amounts, and the geographic adjustment factor, if any, of the revised payment system.

(2) Section 1833(a)(1)(G) of the Act provides that, beginning with the implementation date of a revised payment system for ASC facility services furnished in connection with a surgical procedure pursuant to section 1833(i)(1)(A) of the Act, the amount paid shall be 80 percent of the lesser of the actual charge for such services or the amount determined by the Secretary under the revised payment system.

(3) Section 1833(i)(1)(A) of the Act requires the Secretary to specify the surgical procedures that can be performed safely on an ambulatory basis in an ASC.

(4) Section 1834(d) of the Act specifies that, when screening colonoscopies or screening flexible sigmoidoscopies are performed in an ASC or hospital outpatient department, payment shall be based on the lesser of the amount under the fee schedule that would apply to such services if they were performed in a hospital outpatient department in an area or the amount under the fee schedule that would apply to such services if they were performed in an ambulatory surgical center in the same area. Section 1834(d) of the Act also specifies that, in the case of screening flexible sigmoidoscopy and screening colonoscopy services, the payment amounts must not exceed the payment rates established for the related diagnostic services.

(5) Section 1833(a)(1) of the Act requires 100 percent payment for preventive services described in section 1861(ww)(2) of the Act (excluding electrocardiograms) to which the United States Preventive Services Task Force (USPSTF) has given a grade of A or B for any indication or population. Section 1833(b)(1) of the Act also specifies that the Part B deductible shall not apply with respect to preventive services described in section 1861(ww)(2) of the Act (excluding electrocardiograms) to which the USPSTF has given a grade of A or B for any indication or population.

(b) Scope. This subpart sets forth—

(1) The scope of ASC services and the criteria for determining the covered surgical procedures for which Medicare provides payment for the associated facility services and covered ancillary services;

(2) The basis of payment for facility services and for covered ancillary services furnished in an ASC in connection with a covered surgical procedure;

(3) The methodologies by which Medicare determines payment amounts for ASC services.

[72 FR 42545, Aug. 2, 2007, as amended at 75 FR 72264, Nov. 24, 2010; 77 FR 68558, Nov. 15, 2012]

§416.161 Applicability of this subpart.

The provisions of this subpart apply to ASC services furnished on or after January 1, 2008.

§416.163 General rules.

(a) Payment is made under this subpart for ASC services specified in §§416.164(a) and (b) furnished to Medicare beneficiaries by a participating ASC in connection with covered surgical procedures as determined by the Secretary in accordance with §416.166.

(b) Payment for physicians' services and payment for anesthetists' services are made in accordance with part 414 of this subchapter.

(c) Payment for items and services other than physicians' and anesthetists' services, as specified in §416.164(c), is made in accordance with §410.152 of this subchapter.

§416.164   Scope of ASC services.

(a) Included facility services. ASC services for which payment is packaged into the ASC payment for a covered surgical procedure under §416.166 include, but are not limited to—

(1) Nursing, technician, and related services;

(2) Use of the facility where the surgical procedures are performed;

(3) Any laboratory testing performed under a Clinical Laboratory Improvement Amendments of 1988 (CLIA) certificate of waiver;

(4) Drugs and biologicals for which separate payment is not allowed under the hospital outpatient prospective payment system (OPPS);

(5) Medical and surgical supplies not on pass-through status under subpart G of part 419 of this subchapter;

(6) Equipment;

(7) Surgical dressings;

(8) Implanted prosthetic devices, including intraocular lenses (IOLs), and related accessories and supplies not on pass-through status under subpart G of part 419 of this subchapter;

(9) Implanted DME and related accessories and supplies not on pass-through status under subpart G of part 419 of this subchapter;

(10) Splints and casts and related devices;

(11) Radiology services for which separate payment is not allowed under the OPPS and other diagnostic tests or interpretive services that are integral to a surgical procedure, except certain diagnostic tests for which separate payment is allowed under the OPPS;

(12) Administrative, recordkeeping and housekeeping items and services;

(13) Materials, including supplies and equipment for the administration and monitoring of anesthesia; and

(14) Supervision of the services of an anesthetist by the operating surgeon.

(b) Covered ancillary services. Ancillary items and services that are integral to a covered surgical procedure, as defined in §416.166, and for which separate payment is allowed include:

(1) Brachytherapy sources;

(2) Certain implantable items that have pass-through status under the OPPS;

(3) Certain items and services that CMS designates as contractor-priced, including, but not limited to, the procurement of corneal tissue for corneal transplant procedures;

(4) Certain drugs and biologicals for which separate payment is allowed under the OPPS;

(5) Certain radiology services and certain diagnostic tests for which separate payment is allowed under the OPPS.

(c) Excluded services. ASC services do not include items and services outside the scope of ASC services for which payment may be made under part 414 of this subchapter in accordance with §410.152, including, but not limited to—

(1) Physicians' services (including surgical procedures and all preoperative and postoperative services that are performed by a physician);

(2) Anesthetists' services;

(3) Radiology services (other than those integral to performance of a covered surgical procedure);

(4) Diagnostic procedures (other than those directly related to performance of a covered surgical procedure);

(5) Ambulance services;

(6) Leg, arm, back, and neck braces other than those that serve the function of a cast or splint;

(7) Artificial limbs;

(8) Nonimplantable prosthetic devices and DME.

[72 FR 42545, Aug. 2, 2007, as amended at 79 FR 67030, Nov. 10, 2014; 80 FR 70604, Nov. 13, 2015]

§416.166 Covered surgical procedures.

(a) Covered surgical procedures. Effective for services furnished on or after January 1, 2008, covered surgical procedures are those procedures that meet the general standards described in paragraph (b) of this section (whether commonly furnished in an ASC or a physician's office) and are not excluded under paragraph (c) of this section.

(b) General standards. Subject to the exclusions in paragraph (c) of this section, covered surgical procedures are surgical procedures specified by the Secretary and published in the Federal Register and/or via the Internet on the CMS Web site that are separately paid under the OPPS, that would not be expected to pose a significant safety risk to a Medicare beneficiary when performed in an ASC, and for which standard medical practice dictates that the beneficiary would not typically be expected to require active medical monitoring and care at midnight following the procedure.

(c) General exclusions. Notwithstanding paragraph (b) of this section, covered surgical procedures do not include those surgical procedures that—

(1) Generally result in extensive blood loss;

(2) Require major or prolonged invasion of body cavities;

(3) Directly involve major blood vessels;

(4) Are generally emergent or life-threatening in nature;

(5) Commonly require systemic thrombolytic therapy;

(6) Are designated as requiring inpatient care under §419.22(n) of this subchapter;

(7) Can only be reported using a CPT unlisted surgical procedure code; or

(8) Are otherwise excluded under §411.15 of this subchapter.

[72 FR 42545, Aug. 2, 2007, as amended at 76 FR 74582, Nov. 30, 2011]

§416.167   Basis of payment.

(a) Unit of payment. Under the ASC payment system, prospectively determined amounts are paid for ASC services furnished to Medicare beneficiaries in connection with covered surgical procedures. Covered surgical procedures and covered ancillary services are identified by codes established under the Healthcare Common Procedure Coding System (HCPCS). The unadjusted national payment rate is determined according to the methodology described in §416.171. The manner in which the Medicare payment amount and the beneficiary coinsurance amount for each ASC service is determined is described in §416.172.

(b) Ambulatory payment classification (APC) groups and payment weights. (1) ASC covered surgical procedures are classified using the APC groups described in §419.31 of this subchapter.

(2) For purposes of calculating ASC national payment rates under the methodology described in §416.171, except as specified in paragraph (b)(3) of this section, an ASC relative payment weight is determined based on the APC relative payment weight for each covered surgical procedure and covered ancillary service that has an applicable APC relative payment weight described in §419.31 of this subchapter.

(3) Notwithstanding paragraph (b)(2) of this section, the relative payment weights for services paid in accordance with §416.171(d) are determined so that the national ASC payment rate does not exceed the unadjusted nonfacility practice expense amount paid under the Medicare physician fee schedule for such procedures under subpart B of part 414 of this subchapter.

§416.171 Determination of payment rates for ASC services.

(a) Standard methodology. The standard methodology for determining the national unadjusted payment rate for ASC services is to calculate the product of the applicable conversion factor and the relative payment weight established under §416.167(b), unless otherwise indicated in this section.

(1) Conversion factor for CY 2008. CMS calculates a conversion factor so that payment for ASC services furnished in CY 2008 would result in the same aggregate amount of expenditures as would be made if the provisions in this Subpart F did not apply, as estimated by CMS.

(2) Conversion factor for CY 2009 and subsequent calendar years. The conversion factor for a calendar year is equal to the conversion factor calculated for the previous year, updated as follows:

(i) For CY 2009, the update is equal to zero percent.

(ii) For CY 2010 and subsequent calendar years, the update is the Consumer Price Index for All Urban Consumers (U.S. city average) as estimated by the Secretary for the 12-month period ending with the midpoint of the year involved.

(iii) For CY 2014 and subsequent calendar years, the Consumer Price Index for All Urban Consumers update determined under paragraph (a)(2)(ii) of this section is reduced by 2.0 percentage points for an ASC that fails to meet the standards for reporting of ASC quality measures as established by the Secretary for the corresponding calendar year.

(iv) Productivity adjustment. (A) For calendar year 2011 and subsequent years, the Consumer Price Index for All Urban Consumers determined under paragraph (a)(2)(ii) of this section, after application of any reduction under paragraph (a)(2)(iii) of this section, is reduced by the productivity adjustment described in section 1886(b)(3)(B)(xi)(II) of the Act.

(B) The application of the provisions of paragraph (a)(2)(iv)(A) of this section may result in the update being less than zero percent for a year, and may result in payment rates for a year being less than the payment rates for the preceding year.

(b) Exception. The national ASC payment rates for the following items and services are not determined in accordance with paragraph (a) of this section but are paid an amount derived from the payment rate for the equivalent item or service set under the payment system established in part 419 of this subchapter as updated annually in the Federal Register and/or via the Internet on the CMS Web site. If a payment rate is not available, the following items and services are designated as contractor-priced:

(1) Covered ancillary services specified in §416.164(b), with the exception of radiology services and certain diagnostic tests as provided in §416.164(b)(5);

(2) The device portion of device-intensive procedures, which are procedures with a HCPCS code-level device offset of greater than 40 percent when calculated according to the standard OPPS APC rate setting methodology.

(3) Procedures using certain separately paid implantable devices that are approved for transitional pass-through payment in accordance with §419.66 of this subchapter.

(c) Transitional payment rates. (1) ASC payment rates for CY 2008 are a transitional blend of 75 percent of the CY 2007 ASC payment rate for a covered surgical procedure on the CY 2007 ASC list of surgical procedures and 25 percent of the payment rate for the procedure calculated under the methodology described in paragraph (a) of this section.

(2) ASC payment rates for CY 2009 are a transitional blend of 50 percent of the CY 2007 ASC payment rate for a covered surgical procedure on the CY 2007 ASC list of surgical procedures and 50 percent of the payment rate for the procedure calculated under the methodology described in paragraph (a) of this section.

(3) ASC payment rates for CY 2010 are a transitional blend of 25 percent of the CY 2007 ASC payment rate for a covered surgical procedure on the CY 2007 ASC list of surgical procedures and 75 percent of the payment rate for the procedure calculated under the methodology described in paragraph (a) of this section.

(4) The national ASC payment rate for CY 2011 and subsequent calendar years for a covered surgical procedure designated in accordance with §416.166 is the payment rates for the procedure calculated under the methodology described in paragraph (a) of this section.

(5) Covered ancillary services described in §416.164(b) and surgical procedures identified as covered when performed in an ASC under §416.166 for the first time beginning on or after January 1, 2008, are not subject to the transitional payment rates applicable in CYs 2008 through 2010 for ASC facility services.

(d) Limitation on payment rates for office-based surgical procedures and covered ancillary radiology services and certain diagnostic tests. Notwithstanding the provisions of paragraph (a) of this section, for any covered surgical procedure under §416.166 that CMS determines is commonly performed in physicians' offices or for any covered ancillary radiology service or diagnostic test under §416.164(b)(5), excluding those listed in paragraphs (d)(1) and (d)(2) of this section, the national unadjusted ASC payment rates for these procedures and services will be the lesser of the amount determined under paragraph (a) of this section or the amount calculated at the nonfacility practice expense relative value units under §414.22(b)(5)(i)(B) of this chapter multiplied by the conversion factor described in §414.20(a)(3) of this chapter.

(1) The national unadjusted ASC payment rate for covered ancillary radiology services that involve certain nuclear medicine procedures will be the amount determined under paragraph (a) of this section.

(2) The national unadjusted ASC payment rate for covered ancillary radiology services that use contrast agents will be the amount determined under paragraph (a) of this section.

(e) Budget neutrality. (1) For CY 2008, CMS establishes the conversion factor to result in budget neutrality as estimated by CMS in accordance with paragraph (a)(1) of this section.

(2) For CY 2009 and subsequent calendar years, CMS adjusts the ASC relative payment weights under §416.167(b)(2) as needed so that any updates and adjustments made under §419.50(a) of this subchapter are budget neutral as estimated by CMS.

[72 FR 42545, Aug. 2, 2007, as amended at 75 FR 72264, Nov. 24, 2010; 76 FR 74582, Nov. 30, 2011; 77 FR 277, Jan. 4, 2012; 77 FR 68558, Nov. 15, 2012; 79 FR 67030, Nov. 10, 2014; 81 FR 79879, Nov. 14, 2016]

§416.172   Adjustments to national payment rates.

(a) General rule. Contractors adjust the payment rates established for ASC services to determine Medicare program payment and beneficiary coinsurance amounts in accordance with paragraphs (b) through (g) of this section.

(b) Lesser of actual charge or geographically adjusted payment rate. Payments to ASCs equal 80 percent of the lesser of—

(1) The actual charge for the service; or

(2) The geographically adjusted payment rate determined under this subpart.

(c) Geographic adjustment—(1) General rule. Except as provided in paragraph (c)(2) of this section, the national ASC payment rates established under §416.171 for covered surgical procedures are adjusted for variations in ASC labor costs across geographic areas using wage index values, labor and nonlabor percentages, and localities specified by the Secretary.

(2) Exception. The geographic adjustment is not applied to the payment rates set for drugs, biologicals, devices with OPPS transitional pass-through payment status, and brachytherapy sources.

(d) Deductibles and coinsurance. Part B deductible and coinsurance amounts apply as specified in §§410.152(a) and (i)(2) of this subchapter.

(e) Payment reductions for multiple surgical procedures—(1) General rule. Except as provided in paragraph (e)(2) of this section, when more than one covered surgical procedure for which payment is made under the ASC payment system is performed during an operative session, the Medicare program payment amount and the beneficiary coinsurance amount are based on—

(i) 100 percent of the applicable ASC payment amount for the procedure with the highest national unadjusted ASC payment rate; and

(ii) 50 percent of the applicable ASC payment amount for all other covered surgical procedures.

(2) Exception: Procedures not subject to multiple procedure discounting. CMS may apply any policies or procedures used with respect to multiple procedures under the prospective payment system for hospital outpatient department services under Part 419 of this subchapter as may be consistent with the equitable and efficient administration of this part.

(f) Interrupted procedures. (1) Subject to the provisions of paragraph (f)(2) of this section, when a covered surgical procedure or covered ancillary service is terminated prior to completion due to extenuating circumstances or circumstances that threaten the well-being of the patient, the Medicare program payment amount and the beneficiary coinsurance amount are based on one of the following—

(i) The full program and beneficiary coinsurance amounts if the procedure for which anesthesia is planned is discontinued after the induction of anesthesia or after the procedure is started;

(ii) One-half of the full program and beneficiary coinsurance amounts if the procedure for which anesthesia is planned is discontinued after the patient is prepared for surgery and taken to the room where the procedure is to be performed but before the anesthesia is induced; or

(iii) One-half of the full program and beneficiary coinsurance amounts if a covered surgical procedure or covered ancillary service for which anesthesia is not planned is discontinued after the patient is prepared and taken to the room where the service is to be provided.

(2) Beginning CY 2016, if the covered surgical procedure is a device-intensive procedure, the full device portion of the ASC device-intensive procedure is removed prior to determining the Medicare program payment amount and the beneficiary coinsurance amount identified in paragraph (f)(1)(ii) of this section.

(g) Payment adjustment for new technology intraocular lenses (NTIOLs). A payment adjustment will be made for insertion of an IOL approved as belonging to a class of NTIOLs as defined in subpart G.

[72 FR 42545, Aug. 2, 2007, as amended at 80 FR 70604, Nov. 13, 2015]

§416.173 Publication of revised payment methodologies and payment rates.

CMS publishes annually, through notice and comment rulemaking in the Federal Register and/or via the Internet on the CMS Web site, the payment methodologies and payment rates for ASC services and designates the covered surgical procedures and covered ancillary services for which CMS will make an ASC payment and other revisions as appropriate.

[76 FR 74582, Nov. 30, 2011]

§416.178 Limitations on administrative and judicial review.

There is no administrative or judicial review under section 1869 of the Act, section 1878 of the Act, or otherwise of the following:

(a) The classification system;

(b) Relative weights;

(c) Payment amounts; and

(d) Geographic adjustment factors.

§416.179 Payment and coinsurance reduction for devices replaced without cost or when full or partial credit is received.

(a) General rule. CMS reduces the amount of payment for a covered surgical procedure for which CMS determines that a significant portion of the payment is attributable to the cost of an implanted device not on pass-through status under subpart G of part 419 of this subchapter when one of the following situations occur:

(1) The device is replaced without cost to the ASC or the beneficiary;

(2) The ASC receives full credit for the cost of a replaced device; or

(3) The ASC receives partial credit for the cost of a replaced device but only where the amount of the device credit is greater than or equal to 50 percent of the cost of the new replacement device being implanted.

(b) Amount of reduction to the ASC payment for the covered surgical procedure. (1) The amount of the reduction to the ASC payment made under paragraphs (a)(1) and (a)(2) of this section is calculated in the same manner as the device payment reduction that would be applied to the ASC payment for the covered surgical procedure in order to remove predecessor device costs so that the ASC payment amount for a device with pass-through status under §419.66 of this subchapter represents the full cost of the device, and no packaged device payment is provided through the ASC payment for the covered surgical procedure.

(2) The amount of the reduction to the ASC payment made under paragraph (a)(3) of this section is 50 percent of the payment reduction that would be calculated under paragraph (b)(1) of this section.

(c) Amount of beneficiary coinsurance. The beneficiary coinsurance is calculated based on the ASC payment for the covered surgical procedure after application of the reduction under paragraph (b) of this section.

[72 FR 42545, Aug. 2, 2007, as amended at 72 FR 66932, No. 27, 2007]

Subpart G—Adjustment in Payment Amounts for New Technology Intraocular Lenses Furnished by Ambulatory Service Centers

Source: 71 FR 68226, Nov. 24, 2006, unless otherwise noted.

§416.180   Basis and scope.

(a) Basis. This subpart implements section 141 of Public Law 103-432, which provides for adjustments to payment amounts for new technology intraocular lenses (IOLs) furnished at ambulatory surgical centers (ASCs).

(b) Scope. This subpart sets forth—

(1) The process for interested parties to request that CMS review the appropriateness of the ASC facility fee for insertion of an IOL. This process includes a review of whether that payment is reasonable and related to the cost of acquiring a lens determined by CMS as belonging to a class of new technology IOLs;

(2) Factors that CMS considers for determination of a new class of new technology IOLs; and

(3) Application of the payment adjustment.

§416.185   Process for establishing a new class of new technology IOLs.

(a) Announcement of deadline for requests for review. CMS announces the deadline for each year's requests for review of a new class of new technology IOLs in the final rule updating the ASC payment rates for that calendar year.

(b) Announcement of new classes of new technology IOLs for which review requests have been made and solicitation of public comments. CMS announces the requests for review received in a calendar year and the deadline for public comments regarding the requests in the proposed rule updating the ASC payment rates for the following calendar year. The deadline for submission of public comments is 30 days following the date of the publication of the proposed rule.

(c) Announcement of determinations regarding requests for review. CMS announces its determinations for a calendar year in the final rule updating the ASC payment rates for the following calendar year. CMS publishes the codes and effective dates allowed for those lenses recognized by CMS as belonging to a class of new technology IOLs. New classes of new technology IOLs are effective 30 days following the date of publication of the final rule.

§416.190   Request for review of payment amount.

(a) When requests can be submitted. A request for review of the appropriateness of ASC payment for insertion of an IOL that might qualify for a payment adjustment as belonging to a new class of new technology IOLs must be submitted to CMS in accordance with the annual published deadline.

(b) Who may submit a request. Any individual, partnership, corporation, association, society, scientific or academic establishment, or professional or trade organization able to furnish the information required in paragraph (c) of this section may request that CMS review the appropriateness of the payment amount provided under section 1833(i)(2)(A)(iii) of the Act with respect to an IOL that meets the criteria of a new technology IOL under §416.195.

(c) Content of a request. In order to be accepted by CMS for review, a request for review of the ASC payment amount for insertion of an IOL must include all the information as specified by CMS.

(d) Confidential information. In order for CMS to invoke the protection allowed under Exemption 4 of the Freedom of Information Act (5 U.S.C. 552(b)(4)) and, with respect to trade secrets, the Trade Secrets Act (18 U.S.C. 1905), the requestor must clearly identify all information that is to be characterized as confidential.

§416.195 Determination of membership in new classes of new technology IOLs.

(a) Factors to be considered. CMS uses the following criteria to determine whether an IOL qualifies for a payment adjustment as a member of a new class of new technology IOLs when inserted at an ASC:

(1) The IOL is considered new. CMS will evaluate an application for a new technology IOL only if the IOL type has received initial FDA premarket approval within 3 years prior to the new technology IOL application submission date.

(2) The IOL shall have a new lens characteristic in comparison to currently available IOLs. The labeling, which must be approved by FDA, shall contain a claim of a specific clinical benefit imparted by the new lens characteristic.

(3) The IOL is not described by an active or expired class of new technology IOLs; that is, it does not share a predominant, class-defining characteristic associated with improved clinical outcomes with members of an active or expired class.

(4) Any specific clinical benefit referred to in paragraph (a)(2) of this section must be supported by evidence that demonstrates that the IOL results in a measurable, clinically meaningful, improved outcome. Improved outcomes include:

(i) Reduced risk of intraoperative or postoperative complication or trauma;

(ii) Accelerated postoperative recovery;

(iii) Reduced induced astigmatism;

(iv) Improved postoperative visual acuity;

(v) More stable postoperative vision;

(vi) Other comparable clinical advantages.

(b) CMS determination of eligibility for payment adjustment. CMS reviews the information submitted with a completed request for review, public comments submitted timely, and other pertinent information and makes a determination as follows:

(1) The IOL is eligible for a payment adjustment as a member of a new class of new technology IOLs.

(2) The IOL is a member of an active class of new technology IOLs and is eligible for a payment adjustment for the remainder of the period established for that class.

(3) The IOL does not meet the criteria for designation as a new technology IOL and a payment adjustment is not appropriate.

[71 FR 68226, Nov. 24, 2006, as amended at 77 FR 68558, Nov. 15, 2012; 80 FR 70604, Nov. 13, 2015]

§416.200   Payment adjustment.

(a) CMS establishes the amount of the payment adjustment for classes of new technology IOLs through proposed and final rulemaking in connection with ASC facility services.

(b) CMS adjusts the payment for insertion of an IOL approved as belonging to a class of new technology IOLs for the 5-year period of time established for that class.

(c) Upon expiration of the 5-year period of the payment adjustment, payment reverts to the standard rate for IOL insertion procedures performed in ASCs.

(d) ASCs that furnish an IOL designated by CMS as belonging to a class of new technology IOLs must submit claims using billing codes specified by CMS to receive the new technology IOL payment adjustment

Subpart H—Requirements Under the Ambulatory Surgical Center Quality Reporting (ASCQR) Program

Source: 80 FR 70604, Nov. 13, 2015, unless otherwise noted.

§416.300 Basis and scope of subpart.

(a) Statutory basis. Section 1833(i)(2)(D)(iv) and (i)(7) of the Act authorizes the Secretary to implement a revised ASC payment system in a manner so as to provide for a 2.0 percentage point reduction in any annual update for an ASC's failure to report on quality measures in accordance with the Secretary's requirements.

(b) Scope. This subpart contains specific requirements and standards for the ASCQR Program.

§416.305 Participation and withdrawal requirements under the ASCQR Program.

(a) Participation in the ASCQR Program. Except as provided in paragraph (c) of this section, an ambulatory surgical center (ASC) is considered as participating in the ASCQR Program on the ASC submits any quality measure data to the ASCQR Program and has been designated as open in the Certification and Survey Provider Enhanced Reporting system for at least four months prior to the beginning of data collection for a payment determination.

(b) Withdrawal from the ASCQR Program, (1) An ASC may withdraw from the ASCQR Program by submitting to CMS a withdrawal of participation form that can be found in the secure portion of the QualityNet Web site.

(2) An ASC may withdraw from the ASCQR Program any time up to and including August 31 of the year preceding a payment determination.

(3) Except as provided in paragraph (c) of this section, an ASC will incur a 2.0 percentage point reduction in its ASC annual payment update for that payment determination year and any subsequent payment determinations in which it is withdrawn.

(4) An ASC will be considered as rejoining the ASCQR Program if it begins to submit any quality measure data again to the ASCQR Program.

(c) Minimum case volume for program participation. ASCs with fewer than 240 Medicare claims (Medicare primary and secondary payer) per year during an annual reporting period for a payment determination year are not required to participate in the ASCQR Program for the subsequent annual reporting period for that subsequent payment determination year.

(d) Indian Health Service hospital outpatient department participation. Beginning with the CY 2017 payment determination, Indian Health Service hospital outpatient departments that bill Medicare under the Ambulatory Surgical Center payment system are not considered ASCs for the purposes of the ASCQR Program.

These facilities are not required to meet ASCQR Program requirements and will not receive payment reductions under the ASCQR Program.

§416.310 Data collection and submission requirements under the ASCQR Program.

(a) Requirements for claims-based measures using quality data codes (QDCs). (1) ASCs must submit complete data on individual claims-based quality measures through a claims-based reporting mechanism by submitting the appropriate QDCs on the ASC's Medicare claims.

(2) The data collection period for claims-based quality measures reported using QDCs is the calendar year 2 years prior to the payment determination year. Only claims for services furnished in each calendar year paid by the Medicare Administrative Contractor (MAC) by April 30 of the following year of the ending data collection time period will be included in the data used for the payment determination year.

(3) For ASCQR Program purposes, data completeness for claims-based measures using QDCs is determined by comparing the number of Medicare claims (where Medicare is the primary or secondary payer) meeting measure specifications that contain the appropriate QDCs with the number of Medicare claims that meet measure specifications, but do not have the appropriate QDCs on the submitted Medicare claim. The minimum threshold for successful reporting is that at least 50 percent of Medicare claims meeting measure specifications contain the appropriate QDCs. ASCs that meet this minimum threshold are regarded as having provided complete data for the claims-based measures using QDCs for the ASCQR Program.

(b) Requirements for claims-based measures not using QDCs. The data collection period for claims-based quality measures not using QDCs is paid Medicare fee-for-service claims from the calendar year 2 years prior to the payment determination year. Only claims for services furnished in each calendar year paid by the MAC by April 30 of the following year of the ending data collection time period will be included in the data used for the payment determination.

(c) Requirements for data submitted via an online data submission tool—(1) Requirements for data submitted via a CMS online data submission tool—(i) QualityNet account for Web-based measures. ASCs must maintain a QualityNet account in order to submit quality measure data to the QualityNet Web site for all Web-based measures submitted via a CMS online data submission too. A QualityNet security administrator is necessary to set-up such an account for the purpose of submitting this information.

(ii) Data collection requirements. The data collection time period for quality measures for which data are submitted via a CMS online data submission tool is for services furnished during the calendar year 2 years prior to the payment determination year. Beginning with the CY 2017 payment determination year, data collected must be submitted during the time period of January 1 to May 15 in the year prior to the payment determination year.

(2) Requirements for data submitted via a non-CMS online data submission tool. The data collection time period for ASC-8: Influenza Vaccination Coverage Among Healthcare Personnel is from October 1 of the year 2 years prior to the payment determination year to March 31 during the year prior to the payment determination year. Data collected must be submitted by May 15 in the year prior to the payment determination year.

(d) Extension or exemption. CMS may grant an extension or exemption for the submission of information in the event of extraordinary circumstances beyond the control of an ASC, or a systematic problem with one of CMS' data collection systems directly or indirectly affects data submission. CMS may grant an extension or exemption as follows:

(1) Upon request of the ASC. ASCs may request an extension or exemption within 90 days of the date that the extraordinary circumstance occurred. Specific requirements for submission of a request for an extension or exemption are available on the QualityNet Web site; or

(2) At the discretion of CMS. CMS may grant extensions or exemptions to ASCs that have not requested them when CMS determines that an extraordinary circumstance has occurred.

(e) Requirements for Outpatient and Ambulatory Surgery Consumer Assessment of Healthcare Providers and Systems (OAS CAHPS) Survey. OAS CAHPS is the Outpatient and Ambulatory Surgical Center Consumer Assessment of Healthcare Providers and Systems survey that measures patient experience of care after a recent surgery or procedure at either a hospital outpatient department or an ambulatory surgical center. Ambulatory surgical centers must use an approved OAS CAHPS survey vendor to administer and submit OAS CAHPS data to CMS.

(1) [Reserved]

(2) CMS approves an application for an entity to administer the OAS CAHPS survey as a vendor on behalf of one or more ambulatory surgical centers when the applicant has met the Minimum Survey Requirements and Rules of Participation that can be found on the official OAS CAHPS Web site, and agrees to comply with the current survey administration protocols that can be found on the official OAS CAHPS Web site. An entity must be

approved OAS CAHPS Survey vendor in order to administer the OAS CAHPS Survey and submit data to CMS on behalf of one or more ambulatory surgical centers.

[80 FR 70604, Nov. 13, 2015, as amended at 81 FR 79879, Nov. 14, 2016]

§416.315 Public reporting of data under the ASCQR Program.

Data that an ASC submitted for the ASCQR Program will be made publicly available on a CMS Web site after providing the ASC an opportunity to review the data to be made public. CMS will publicly display ASC data by the National Provider Identifier (NPI) when data are submitted by the NPI. CMS will publicly display ASC data by the CMS Certification Number (CCN) when data are submitted by the CCNs.

§416.320 Retention and removal of quality measures under the ASCQR Program.

(a) General rule for the retention of quality measures. Quality measures adopted for an ASCQR Program measure set for a previous payment determination year are retained in the ASCQR Program for measure sets for subsequent payment determination years, except when they are removed, suspended, or replaced as set forth in paragraphs (b) and (c) of this section.

(b) Immediate measure removal. In cases where CMS believes that the continued use of a measure as specified raises patient safety concerns, CMS will immediately remove a quality measure from the ASCQR Program and will promptly notify ASCs and the public of the removal of the measure and the reasons for its removal through the ASCQR Program ListServ and the ASCQR Program

QualityNet Web site. CMS will confirm the removal of the measure for patient safety concerns in the next ASCQR Program rulemaking.

(c) Measure removal, suspension, or replacement through the rulemaking process. Unless a measure raises specific safety concerns as set forth in paragraph (b) of this section, CMS will use the regular rulemaking process to remove, suspend, or replace quality measures in the ASCQR Program to allow for public comment.

(1) Criteria for removal of quality measures. (i) CMS will use the following criteria to determine whether to remove a measure from the ASCQR Program:

(A) Measure performance among ASCs is so high and unvarying that meaningful distinctions and improvements in performance can no longer be made (topped-out measures);

(B) Availability of alternative measures with a stronger relationship to patient outcomes;

(C) A measure does not align with current clinical guidelines or practice;

(D) The availability of a more broadly applicable (across settings, populations, or conditions) measure for the topic;

(E) The availability of a measure that is more proximal in time to desired patient outcomes for the particular topic;

(F) The availability of a measure that is more strongly associated with desired patient outcomes for the particular topic; and

(G) Collection or public reporting of a measure leads to negative unintended consequences other than patient harm.

(ii) The benefits of removing a measure from the ASCQR Program will be assessed on a case-by-case basis. A measure will not be removed solely on the basis of meeting any specific criterion.

(2) Criteria to determine topped-out measures. For the purposes of the ASCQR Program, a measure is considered to be topped-out under paragraph (c)(1)(i)(A) of this section when it meets both of the following criteria:

(i) Statistically indistinguishable performance at the 75th and 90th percentiles (defined as when the difference between the 75th and 90th percentiles for an ASC's measure is within two times the standard error of the full data set); and

(ii) A truncated coefficient of variation less than or equal to 0.10.

§416.325   Measure maintenance under the ASCQR Program.

(a) Measure maintenance under the ASCQR Program. CMS follows different procedures to update the measure specifications under the ASCQR Program based on whether the change is substantive or nonsubstantive. CMS will determine what constitutes a substantive versus a nonsubstantive change to a measure's specifications on a case-by-case basis.

(b) Substantive changes. CMS will continue to use rulemaking to adopt substantive updates to measures in the ASCQR Program.

(c) Nonsubstantive changes. If CMS determines that a change to a measure previously adopted in the ASCQR Program is nonsubstantive, CMS will use a subregulatory process to revise the ASCQR Program Specifications Manual so that it clearly identifies the changes to that measure and provide links to where additional information on the changes can be found. When a measure undergoes subregulatory maintenance, CMS will provide notification of the measure specification update on the QualityNet Web site and in the ASCQR Program Specifications Manual, and will provide sufficient lead time for ASCs to implement the revisions where changes to the data collection systems would be necessary.

§416.330 Reconsiderations under the ASCQR Program.

(a) Reconsiderations of ASCQR Program decisions. An ASC may request reconsideration of a decision by CMS that it has not met the requirements of the ASCQR Program for a particular payment determination year. An ASC must submit a reconsideration request to CMS by no later than the first business day on or after March 17 of the affected payment year.

(b) Requirements for reconsideration requests. A reconsideration request must contain the following information:

(1) The ASC CCN and related NPI(s);

(2) The name of the ASC;

(3) The CMS-identified reason for not meeting the requirements of the ASCQR Program for the affected payment determination year as provided in any CMS notification to the ASC;

(4) The ASC's basis for requesting reconsideration. The ASC must identify its specific reason(s) for believing it met the ASCQR Program requirements for the affected payment determination year and should not be subject to the reduced ASC annual payment update;

(5) The ASC-designated personnel contact information, including name, email address, telephone number, and mailing address (must include physical mailing address, not just a post office box); and

(6) A copy of all materials that the ASC submitted to comply with the requirements of the affected ASCQR Program payment determination year. With regard to information on claims, ASCs are not required to submit copies of all submitted claims, but instead may focus on the specific claims at issue. For these claims, ASCs should submit relevant information, which could include copies of the actual claims at issue.

(c) Reconsideration process. Upon receipt of a request for reconsideration, CMS will do the following:

(1) Provide an email acknowledgement, using the contact information provided in the reconsideration request, notifying the ASC that the request has been received; and

(2) Provide a formal response to the ASC contact using the information provided in the reconsideration request notifying the ASC of the outcome of the reconsideration process.

(d) Final ASCQR Program payment determination. For an ASC that submits a timely reconsideration request, the reconsideration determination is the final ASCQR Program payment determination. For an ASC that does not submit a timely reconsideration request, the CMS determination is the final payment determination. There is no appeal of any final ASCQR Program payment determination.

Source:

The Conditions for Coverage can be accessed on line at the Electronic Code of Federal Regulations web site for Title 42 – Public Health:

http://www.ecfr.gov/cgi-bin/text-idx?c=ecfr&rgn=div5&view=text&node=42:3.0.1.1.3&idno=42

There are is wealth of information on the internet that you can use to obtain additional information in your role as a board member. Your administrative team should be accessing these sites on a regular basis. For your information, we have provided the following links for you to review research on your own:

CMS Web Site

The CMS web site provides a considerable amount of information about your Medicare certification. Here are links to important information available:

Ambulatory Surgery Center Portal:

https://www.cms.gov/Center/Provider-Type/Ambulatory-Surgical-Centers-ASC-Center.html

Medicare Payment Information:

https://www.cms.gov/Medicare/Medicare-Fee-for-Service-Payment/ASCPayment/index.html

ASC Association

The Ambulatory Surgery Center Association is a nonprofit association that represents all aspects of the Ambulatory Surgery Center industry including the physicians, nurses, administrative staff and owners. The web site provides access to information about all aspects about the industry:

www.ascassociation.org

National Fire Protection Association (NFPA)

According to the NFPA website at www.nfpa.org, "the association delivers information and knowledge through more than 300 consensus codes and standards, research, training, education, outreach and advocacy; and by partnering with others who share an interest in furthering the NFPA mission." All NFPA codes and standards can be viewed on their website for free. To print the standards, you will have to purchase access. You can also buy copies of the published books either through NFPA or an online bookseller.

Note that as of the date of publication of this book, CMS has adopted the 2000 Edition of NFPA 101. It is expected that shortly, CMS will adopt the 2012 Edition.

Association for Professionals in Infection Control and Epidemiology (APIC)

APIC (www.apic.org) is one of the leading sources of infection control standards for the ASC industry. The organization publishes various books and provides regular training programs on infection control.

APIC provides regular training for infection control coordinators in ASCs and it has become the "defacto" standard that these coordinators attend this course.

Association for Operating Room Nurses (AORN)

AORN (www.aorn.org) is one of the most influential societies in the ASC industries and ASCs should encourage operating room staff members to join the organization and become CNOR Certified (Certified Nurse Operating Room).

AORN publishes a variety of books that provide guidance and standards for operating room management. Their educational programs provide training in a variety of areas applicable to ambulatory surgery centers.

Their publication "Guidelines for Perioperative Practice" is the industry's leading guide for operating room standards. Every ASC should maintain a copy of this book.

Certified Ambulatory Surgery Center Credential (CASC)

The CASC credential is overseen by the Board of Ambulatory Surgery Certification (www.aboutcasc.org). Administrators and nursing directors who wish to obtain the CASC credential must undergo a rigorous test to determine their knowledge of the industry and the responsibilities of the chief executive officer of ASCs.

To reduce the risk that the organization hires unqualified individuals, your governing body's may wish to consider hiring administrators that carry the CASC credential.

The Facility Guidelines Institute (FGI)

FGI provides information about the *Guidelines for Design and Construction Health Care Facilities* – the definitive guide for construction standards applicable to healthcare organizations, including ambulatory surgery centers. The web site provides information about the guidelines and links to purchase the official books. Their web site is:

http://www.fgiguidelines.org/index.php

Eden Group Development, Inc.

The publisher of this book and the author maintain a web site where you can purchase books specifically written for the ambulatory surgery center industry at;

http://www.reg-books.com

The books include the best-selling The Survey Guide for ASCs A Guide to the CMS Conditions for Coverage & Interpretive Guidelines for Ambulatory Surgery Centers and Ambulatory Surgery Center Governance - A Guide for Ambulatory Surgery Center Owners & Governing Body Members. These books are important additions to your ASC library and will help you prepare for a survey.

Ambulatory Healthcare Strategies, LLC

The author is also a nationally known consultant and maintains a web site at:

http://www.ah-strategies.com

Ambulatory Healthcare Strategies, LLC (AHS) caters to the Ambulatory Surgery (ASC) and Office-Based Surgery industry. AHS provides a full range of services to meet the administrative, regulatory and financial needs of your organization. AHS is NOT a management company, but provides many of the same services that a traditional management company provides. AHS don't take ownership, and their on-going fees are on a retainer basis with a fixed monthly fee.

Ambulatory Healthcare Strategies provides a unique business model – totally focused on what your organization's needs – not on a "cookie cutter" approach to outsourced services. Their business model provides a variety of outsourced service offerings ranging from one-time consulting services up to on-going retainer-based oversight services.

The AHS monthly fixed retainer-based Regulatory & Accreditation Oversight and Financial Oversight Services are unique to the industry and can often replace existing management company services for a fraction of the cost.

AHS Consulting Services include:

- Responding to State, CMS and Accreditation Surveys (Plan of Correction, Mitigation of Citations, Crisis Management)
- Interim Administrator/Clinical Management Services
- Accreditation and CMS Survey Preparation and Mock Surveys
- Financial Projections and Feasibility Studies
- Policy & Procedure Review and Updates and Maintenance Services
- Business Office, Billing System and Billing Service Reviews

Monthly Retainer Services:

Retainer services are geared specifically to the needs of your organization and the monthly fixed retainer fee is based on the services that you request. AHS does not require long-term contracts and their low overhead assures our fees are considerably less than the same services provided by a management company.

Owners and administrators of surgery centers and office based surgery practices major challenge in keeping up with the constant changes in the regulatory environment. Their retainer services are designed to give you the information and resources you need to keep current – without having to hire full-time compliance staff.

AHS monthly retainers can include:

- Maintenance of your Policy and Procedure Manual
- Oversight of your QI Program
- Attendance at your Committee and Governing Body Meetings and preparation of the agenda and minutes
- Preparation and management of your organizations strategic plan and goals and objectives
- Preparation of Monthly and Quarterly Financial Statements
- Assistance in preparing QI Studies
- State and Federal Reporting
- On-site training and education
- Preparation of budgets and financial projections
- Assistance in ownership transfers and recruitment
- Negotiations of Contracts
- Credentialing and Employee File oversight and electronic file maintenance
- Attendance at Surveys and preparation for upcoming surveys, follow-up after surveys

All retainers include:

- Access to the Surgery Center Academy – an on-line training portal providing employee orientation and annual mandatory education programs prepared specifically for your organization. This can supplement and or replace many of your in-house training programs

- Access to our unique database of educational programs for administrators and managers in your organization
- Annual Mock Survey for compliance with CMS Conditions for Coverage
- On-going text, email and phone access to our staff 24/7.

For more information, visit the AHS web site at www.ah-strategies.com or call John Goehle directly at 585-594-1167.

John J. Goehle is the Chief Operating Officer and partner with Ambulatory Healthcare Strategies, LLC based in Rochester, New York.

John is a Certified Public Accountant licensed in the State of New York and holds a Master's in Business Administration from Heriot-Watt University in Edinburgh, Scotland. He also holds the prestigious Certified Administrator – ASC (CASC) credential.

John is a 27 year veteran of ambulatory surgery centers and a national leader in ASC industry. He is a popular speaker on ASC finance, accounting, budgeting and administration. He has taught college courses in health care finance, economics and information systems. In 2005 he wrote "Finance Management Made Easy – Strategies for Ambulatory Surgery Centers" for HC Pro. In 2008 he wrote "APCs for ASCs Strategies for Success Under the New Payment System", also for HC Pro. He also co-authored both the first and second editions of the ASC Association's (formerly FASA) book "Finance and Accounting for ASC's."

You may contact the author through email at jgoehle@ah-strategies.com.

www.ingramcontent.com/pod-product-compliance
Lightning Source LLC
Chambersburg PA
CBHW071221220526
45468CB00002B/694